Carlos Alberto do Amaral Medeiros
Giulia Luiza Cecconello
Giancarlos Brum Fornari

Sleep disorders in secondary school students

Carlos Alberto do Amaral Medeiros
Giulia Luiza Cecconello
Giancarlos Brum Fornari

Sleep disorders in secondary school students

A portrait of the sleeping habits of public school students in Chapecó, Santa Catarina

Imprint

Any brand names and product names mentioned in this book are subject to trademark, brand or patent protection and are trademarks or registered trademarks of their respective holders. The use of brand names, product names, common names, trade names, product descriptions etc. even without a particular marking in this work is in no way to be construed to mean that such names may be regarded as unrestricted in respect of trademark and brand protection legislation and could thus be used by anyone.

Cover image: www.ingimage.com

This book is a translation from the original published under ISBN 978-613-9-63806-2.

Publisher:
Sciencia Scripts
is a trademark of
Dodo Books Indian Ocean Ltd. and OmniScriptum S.R.L publishing group

120 High Road, East Finchley, London, N2 9ED, United Kingdom
Str. Armeneasca 28/1, office 1, Chisinau MD-2012, Republic of Moldova, Europe
Printed at: see last page
ISBN: 978-620-7-68771-8

ACKNOWLEDGEMENTS

We would like to thank our supervisors Dr Carlos Frederico de Almeida Rodrigues and Mr Carlos Alberto do Amaral Medeiros, who encouraged us to do our work in the best possible way. To the schools in Chapecó who opened their doors to us and to our parents, without whom we would never be here.

SUMMARY

Introduction: Although sleep is a fundamental behavioural state in the physiological maintenance of the body, chronic sleep restriction is becoming increasingly widespread in the population, affecting even adolescents, who are showing a reduction in the amount of time they sleep per night. Among the reasons why young people are getting fewer nights of sleep are anxiety and stress, which are risk factors for sleep disorders. **Objectives: To** analyse the prevalence of sleep-wake cycle disorders in adolescent high school students from public schools in the city of Chapecó-SC. **Methodology:** This is an observational, analytical, cross-sectional study in which data was collected using a questionnaire containing objective and discursive questions and the Pittsburgh Sleep Quality Index (PSQI). **Results:** 276 students were interviewed, 53.99% of whom were students in the second year of secondary school. Analysis of the results showed that 69.20 per cent of the students had poor sleep quality and that 10.87 per cent may have an established sleep disorder.

Conclusion: It can be concluded that sleep disorders among adolescents are a real problem that deserves attention from parents, educators and the medical community in general. According to the findings of this study, the rates of poor sleep-wake cycle quality in the young population were significantly high and independent of gender and grade.

Keywords: sleep; disorder; adolescent

EPIGRAPH

This is the refuge of the unfortunate - the prisoner's release, the soft lap of the disillusioned, the weary, the broken-hearted; of all the delightful functions of nature this is the main one; what happiness for a man when the anxieties and passions of the day are over.

Tristram Shandy

SUMMARY

CHAPTER 1

INTRODUCTION

Man has always sought to understand his sleep-wake cycle, as well as that of other animals. A few centuries ago, this understanding was essential for human survival, as food and protection against nocturnal attacks depended on it (TUFIK, 2008). Closely linked to sleep are dreams, which are still a mystery to mankind today. Dreams have also contributed to the creation of the myths and legends of ancient civilisations. A common thread among these myths is the idea that during sleep, the soul leaves the body, making it immobile and unconscious. Many of these beliefs persist to this day, but with different characteristics (TIMO-IARIA, 2008).

Although sleep is a fundamental behavioural state in the physiological maintenance of the body, chronic sleep restriction is increasingly common in industrialised societies (TUFIK, 2008). This sleep restriction is becoming more and more widespread in the population, even affecting adolescents, who are showing a reduction in sleep time during the week (CARSKADON, apud Beijamini, 2008).

Among the reasons why young people are getting fewer nights of sleep are anxiety and stress, which are risk factors for sleep disorders (ROCHA; ROSSINI; REIMAO, 2010). Adolescents who are attending secondary school go through a period of transition in which these feelings are experienced with great intensity, a factor that can trigger sleep disorders (ALMONDES, 2003). Other reasons that have led adolescents to have bad nights are external factors, such as fixed school hours, going out at night with friends, spending hours awake at night watching television or surfing the internet (ROCHA; ROSSINI; REIMAO, 2010).

The advent of virtual communication platforms and wireless internet also contributes to sleep restriction, as it has profoundly changed the lifestyle habits of young people and adults in the 21st century. It's not uncommon to find teenagers spending sleepless nights in front of their computer or laptop, playing network games against friends or even with people on the other side of the world. The results of these new habits are worrying: excessive daytime sleepiness and afternoon naps have become the norm among young people, and there is another negative implication that worries their parents greatly: a lack of interest in school and everything related to it (DUARTE, 2007).

A poor night's sleep can have a negative impact on the next day's routine, causing damage such as drowsiness, mood fluctuations, anxiety, slow thinking and, consequently, a significant drop in school performance (CIAMPO, 2012).

Therefore, taking these assumptions into account, it would be interesting to assess the prevalence of sleep-wake cycle disorders in high school students from public schools in Chapecó, as well as to compare the prevalence of cases of sleep disorders between grades and identify the influence of gender on the quality of sleep of these young people.

CHAPTER 2

OBJECTIVES

2.1 General objective

To analyse the prevalence of sleep-wake cycle disorders in adolescent high school students from public schools in the city of Chapecó-SC.

2. 2Specific objectives

To evaluate the relationship between sleep disorders and the students' level of education;

To compare sleep quality between genders;

Check the prevalence of late-night use of electronic devices.

CHAPTER 3

THEORETICAL BACKGROUND

3.1 Sleep physiology

Normal sleep is made up of alternating NREM (non-rapid eye movements) and REM (rapid eye movements) stages, which are differentiated by electroencephalogram (EEG) wave patterns, the presence or absence of rapid eye movements and muscle tone (ALOE; AZEVEDO; HASAN, 2005).

NREM sleep is the longest-lasting phase (75 to 80 per cent of all sleep). REM sleep occupies approximately 20 to 25 per cent of sleep time, ranging from five to 30 minutes, recurring every 90 to 110 minutes and its first episode occurs in the second hour of sleep (SANTOS et al., 2014).

In NREM sleep there is muscle relaxation compared to wakefulness, but muscle tone is maintained (FERNANDES, 2006). In REM sleep, there is a loss of muscle tone accompanied by the onset of rapid eye movements and desynchronisation of the EEG (RECHTSHAFFEN, 1968). REM sleep is the last and deepest stage of sleep, but the EEG pattern is the same as if the person were awake. It is during REM sleep that most of the dreams we have during the night occur. Dreams are thought to be involved in synaptic reorganisation and the processing of plastic functions relating to homeostasis in brain areas related to memory, learning and psychic functions (FERNANDES, 2006).

3.2 Sleep disorders

To facilitate the understanding and treatment of sleep disorders, classifications have been postulated, such as the International Classification of Sleep Disorders (ICSD), developed by the American Sleep Disorders Association in 1990, which consists of the classification of disorders that are primarily associated with sleep disturbances, as well as pathological conditions that begin or occur during sleep

(BUYSSE, 2003).

The second edition of the ICSD (ICSD-2), published in 2005 by the American Academy of Sleep Medicine, distributed the more than 90 types of sleep-wake cycle disorders into eight broad categories (insomnia, sleep-related breathing disorders, hypersomnia of central origin not caused by circadian cycle disorders, circadian rhythm sleep disorders, parasomnias, among others), citing their characteristics, diagnosis and treatment proposals (TORPHY, 2012). The first of these is insomnia, considered to be the most common sleep disorder in the population, characterised by difficulty initiating sleep, waking up several times during the night, difficulty getting back to sleep and daytime fatigue. The very tension generated by the need to sleep ends up having a negative effect on sleep, due to the neurological arousal. It's important to make it clear that without associated daytime dysfunction, insomnia cannot be diagnosed. The second category is excessive daytime sleepiness (EDS), diagnosed by the patient's inability to stay awake and alert during the day, even presenting unintentional sleep lapses, the main cause of which is chronic sleep deprivation (NEVES, 2013).

Also included in the new ICSD-2 classification are "abnormal events during sleep" and "REM sleep behaviour disorder". The abnormal events section includes parasomnias (peculiar manifestations and behaviours during sleep, most of which do not constitute an abnormality) and movement disorders (mainly restless legs syndrome). The most frequently diagnosed REM sleep parasomnias are confused waking, sleepwalking, night terrors, REM sleep behaviour disorder and nightmares.

3.3 Main sleep disorders in adolescence

In modern society, sleep disorders, especially insomnia and excessive daytime sleepiness, are the most common complaints in the general population. It is estimated that the prevalence of insomnia in populations ranges from 30 to 50 per cent (TUFIK, 2008) and that excessive daytime sleepiness (EDS) has an approximate prevalence of between 10 and 25 per cent of the general population (GIORELLI, 2012).

The percentage of young adolescents who complain of suffering from some kind of sleep disorder is on average 25% (WANTANABE, 2010), while in the general population this figure varies from 15% to 27% (MULLER; GUIMARÃES, 2007). In a study carried out by Liu et al. (2007) with 1056 adolescents, 18.8 per cent of the adolescents reported poor sleep quality, 26.2 per cent reported not being satisfied with their sleep, 16.1 per cent had insomnia and 17.9 per cent had daytime sleepiness.

3.3.1 Excessive daytime sleepiness

Excessive daytime sleepiness (EDS) is commonly mistaken for a disorder, but it is actually a complex symptom with a variable aetiology. The main causes of EDS include: quantity and quality of sleep, waking time and associated medical or neurological conditions or any medical condition that can impair sleep. The use of psychoactive substances and the presence of primary hypersomnia are also factors that can trigger excessive daytime sleepiness (GIORELLI, 2012).

Adolescence is a phase in which the patterns of the sleep-wake cycle change radically: while children have a more morning-like cycle, young adolescents are biologically programmed to sleep and wake up later. This phenomenon can be explained by medical findings indicating a peak in the volume of the brain's grey matter during adolescence, the grey matter being sensitive to variations in the body, including those related to sleep (CIAMPO, 2012; PEREIRA, 2010).

The greater propensity for excessive daytime sleepiness in adolescents is due to biological, environmental and behavioural factors. The increase in school, extracurricular and social activities has caused changes in sleep patterns during adolescence (PEREIRA, 2010). A determining biological factor is the slowdown in the inhibition of melatonin secretion at the start of the light phase of the day, which occurs mainly in the late stages of puberty, facilitating the occurrence of EDS at this stage of human development (BERNARDO, 2009; PEREIRA, 2010).

EDS is usually rare in adolescents. It is not usually related to poor sleep hygiene, but rather underlies some other disorder, which must be diagnosed and treated appropriately to avoid compromises and impacts on the adolescent's life (ANTUNES; FERNANDES; SILVEIRA, 2013). The possible differential diagnoses of EDS due to poor sleep hygiene can be of various etiologies, such as obstructive sleep apnoea, narcolepsy, restless legs syndrome, drugs and medications and others (CHELLAPPA, 2010).

As its first incidence peaks at the age of 15 (ANTUNES; FERNANDES; SILVEIRA, 2013), the study of narcolepsy is relevant to this study. Narcolepsy is an intrinsic sleep disorder in which there are instabilities in the maintenance of the sleep-wake cycle, the most common symptoms of which are EDS and cataplexy, which may appear years apart (CABRAL et al., 2009). Cataplexy is the name given to one of the characteristic symptoms of narcolepsy, corresponding to muscle weakness, typically bilateral, triggered by an emotional stimulus (RODRIGUES, 2012).Narcolepsy will always be accompanied by excessive daytime sleepiness of varying degrees of severity, while cataplexy will be present in 70% of narcolepsy cases (COELHO et al., 2007).

3.3.2 Insomnia

According to the Brazilian Sleep Society (2003), insomnia is a symptom that can be defined as difficulty in initiating and/or maintaining sleep, the presence of non-restorative sleep, i.e. insufficient to maintain a good quality of alertness and physical and mental well-being during the day, with consequent impairment of performance in daytime activities.

In insomnia, the waking period is always affected, with changes in behaviour and physical disposition, such as tiredness, dejection, adynamia and daytime sleepiness. Mood changes are also recurrent, such as irritability, apathy and inattention (ALVES; EJZENBERG; OKAY, 2002).

According to Halbower and Marcus (2003, apud ROCHA; ROSSINI; REIMAO, 2010), insomnia is a common disorder in adolescence, with an approximate prevalence of 2.2% to 17%. In adolescence, the main causes of insomnia are: phase delay, individual variability (afternoon versus morning), anxiety, family or school pressure, emotional disorders (anorexia, schizophrenia, mania), restless legs syndrome, obstructive sleep apnoea-hypopnoea syndrome and other chronic or acute illnesses (NUNES; CAVALCANTE, 2005).

Insomnia due to changes in the circadian rhythm, known as phase delay, occurs more frequently in adolescence. The condition begins with a tendency to go to sleep later each day (at weekends or on holiday) and consequently wake up later. This situation is often the result of physiological changes that occur in the circadian rhythm during puberty. The initial symptom is difficulty waking up at a routine time in the morning, with afternoon naps on the way home from school (LOUZADA; BARRETO, 2004).

3.3.3 Obstructive sleep apnoea syndrome in childhood and adolescence

Obstructive sleep apnoea syndrome (OSAS) is characterised by episodes of total or partial obstruction of the upper airways during sleep, associated with a drop in oxygen saturation or hypercapnia (NUNES, 2002). The importance of knowledge about the syndrome for this study is clear and indisputable, given that OSAS is one of the most common sleep disorders in adolescence (PETROV; LICHSTEIN; BALDWIN, 2014). Furthermore, people with apnoea often suffer from excessive daytime sleepiness (EDS) resulting from "micro-awakenings" during sleep (MULLER; GUIMARÃES, 2007). The most common signs of OSAS are snoring, excessive sleepiness and breathing pauses during sleep (BITTENCOURT et al., 2009).

OSAS is currently understood to be a relatively common syndrome in childhood and adolescence, with an estimated prevalence of 2% to 3% in developed countries (MOREIRA, 2009). One of the possible causes for the high rate of sleep apnoea in children and adolescents is the increased prevalence of overweight and obesity at increasingly earlier ages (ENES; SLATER, 2010), since obesity is the main risk factor for the syndrome in the adult population, as evidenced by the fact that around two thirds of OSAS patients are obese (BALBANI; FORMIGONI, 1999).

Surgical intervention is indicated in cases where there are anatomical alterations or to help with other treatments (BITTENCOURT et al., 2009). Anatomical alterations such as palatine tonsil hypertrophy are the main cause of OSAS among children and adolescents (MOREIRA, 2009).

3.4 Sleep and learning

Biological and social factors interfere with the change in the chronobiological sleep cycle in adolescents, who start to feel the urge to sleep later and later (LOUZADA et al., 2008). Learning can be affected by the change in the chronobiological cycle, as it depends on memory consolidation, and sleep plays a key role in this process (VALLE; VALLE; REIMÃO, 2009).

Memorisation and logical reasoning are affected by poor quality sleep or sleep deprivation. This is because the information we take in and learn throughout the day is consolidated while we sleep (BOSCOLO, 2007). Without the daily process of the sleep-wake cycle, everyday activities such as working, studying and even driving would become difficult tasks. Sleep promotes memory sedimentation, resting the body and mind by conserving and restoring energy (CARDOSO et al., 2009).

3.5 Sleep-wake cycle and adolescence

As Almondes (2003) states, the sleep-wake cycle is a circadian rhythm, i.e. it is related to environmental factors and oscillates over a 24-hour period. Exogenous and endogenous factors affect the cycle. Exogenous factors include: day-night alternation, school schedules, working hours, leisure time and family activities. Endogenously, the sleep-wake cycle can be regulated by the suprachiasmatic nucleus and other biological rhythms in the body, such as melatonin.

According to Addams, Ropper and Victor (2000), the sleep-wake cycle varies according to the age of individuals. Newborn babies sleep between 16 and 20 hours a day and in childhood between 10 and 12. By the age of 10, sleep time drops to around 9 to 10 hours. Teenagers, on the other hand, usually sleep between 7 and 7.5 hours a night.

Carskadon (1980, apud PEREZ, 2007) suggests that in adolescence there is a need for more than eight hours of sleep per night, but adolescents get fewer hours of sleep than recommended. It's important to emphasise that there are individual differences that can alter the duration and depth of each person's sleep, apparently varying according to genetic factors, neonatal conditions, physical activities and psychological particularities (ADDAMS; ROPPER; VICTOR, 2000).

Some behaviours that characterise young people's lives, such as social activities, lead them to acquire nocturnal habits, while school activities require them to be fully awake early in the morning. Consequently, there is a reduction in sleep time over the course of the week, leading to a vicious cycle of sleep debt (PEREZ-CHADA, 2007).Other factors that lead to a reduction in necessary sleep time, apart from school schedules, are inadequate eating habits (GIBSON et al., 2006), a sedentary lifestyle, too much time watching television or using computers, tablets, mobile phones and derivatives (GAINA et al., 2007) and, especially, entering the world of work (TEIXEIRA et al., 2010). When sleep is restricted, adolescents' behaviour can show signs of changes in mood and behaviour. Aggressiveness, uncontrolled emotional responses, changes in the quality of school performance and inattention are common consequences in individuals with sleep deprivation or poor sleep quality. These signs can worsen and lead to symptoms of hyperactivity, especially in adolescents who are undergoing hormonal changes (FINIMUNDI, 2012).

3.5.1 External factors that can affect sleep quality in adolescents

A study by Bernardo (2009) showed that the main variable associated with less than 8 hours of sleep in adolescents was age. With increasing age, young people showed a decrease in hours of sleep. Another variable analysed was involvement in the world of work, and there was a tendency for sleep duration to decrease among working adolescents in the lower, middle and upper social classes. The school shift and the habit of napping were also found to be variables associated with less than 8 hours of sleep.

Another similar study (TEIXEIRA, 2007), which aimed to assess the sleep and sleepiness of working and non-working evening high school students, found that the average duration of sleep during the week was shorter among workers (7.2 hours) than non-workers (8.8 hours). It was also possible to analyse that during the week and during classes, workers were moderately sleepier than non-workers.

15

CHAPTER 4

METHODOLOGY

4.1 Type of study

This was a descriptive, observational and cross-sectional study. Data was collected using questionnaires containing objective and subjective questions. This is a quantitative exploratory study in which the prevalence of sleep disorders in adolescent high school students from public schools was observed.

4.2 Population and sampling

The entire research sample was made up of teenage students from public schools in the city of Chapecó, who were attending high school and whose parents agreed to their children answering the questionnaire. The population of secondary school students in the city's public schools is 6,326 (six thousand three hundred and twenty-six) individuals. The concept of adolescent adopted by the Ministry of Health in Brazil is the same as that defined by the World Health Organisation (WHO), which establishes the age range of 10 to 19 as the period of adolescence.

The sample required for the study was calculated using EpInfo software, version 7. The percentage of young adolescents who complain of suffering from some kind of sleep disorder is, on average, 25% (WANTANABE, 2010), while in the general population this figure varies from 15% to 27% (MULLER; GUIMARÃES, 2007). This determined a minimum sample of 276 students, with a 95% confidence level.

4.3 Criteria for inclusion and exclusion

4.3.1 Criteria for inclusion

The study included adolescents between 10 and 19 years of age, regularly enrolled in public high schools in the city of Chapecó-SC, in the morning and afternoon shifts. The research subjects were previously authorised by their legal representatives to answer the questionnaire "*Pittsburgh* Sleep Quality Index '>.

4.3.2Criteria   for exclusion

All individuals who did not fall into the 10-19 age bracket and who were not regularly enrolled at the school in question were excluded from the study. Students on the night shift were also excluded, due to a possible bias that would jeopardise the results of the research. Those who did not present a signed informed consent form from their legal guardians were automatically excluded from the study.

4.   4Data collection

Data was collected collectively during the first half of 2016, during class time. The research took place in five of the 19 public schools in the city of Chapecó. In order to choose them, a mapping process was carried out,

dividing the city into five sectors, prioritising the choice of one school for each of these sectors.

To collect the data, an educational approach was given on the importance of getting a good night's sleep, followed by the application of the Pittsburgh Sleep Quality Index (PSQI) questionnaire (APPENDIX I) to students who agreed to answer the questionnaire. The activity was carried out after the Free and Informed Consent Form (APPENDIX I) had been signed by the parents or guardians of the research subjects who were under 18 years of age.

The PSQI has a sensitivity of 89.6% and specificity of 86.5% (BUYSSE et al., 1989). The index is a self-administered questionnaire made up of 10 questions. Questions one, two, three and four are open-ended and questions five to 10 are objective. The questions make up seven components, each of which can vary in score from zero to three points, with the maximum score being 21 (CARDOSO, 2009).

The seven components of the PSQI are: subjective sleep quality, sleep latency, sleep duration, habitual sleep efficiency, sleep disturbances, use of sleep medication and daytime dysfunction (BUYSSE et al., 1989).

A score of more than five points indicates that the individual is experiencing major difficulties in at least two components, or moderate difficulties in more than three components (BERTOLAZI, 2008). Scores of zero to four indicate good sleep quality, five to 10 indicate poor quality and above 10 indicate sleep disturbance (BUYSSE et al., 1989).

Two more questions were added to the PSQI to meet the research objectives (APPENDIX I).

4.5Analysing   and interpreting the results

The data collected from the information systems was analysed using the Statistical Package for Social Sciences (SPSS) version 19.0 ®. The data is

considered statistically significant when the significance level is 5% ($p<0.05$).

When there was a need to compare variables, statistical tests were used according to the type of variable. The chi-squared test (X^2) was used for qualitative variables and *Student's t-test* for quantitative variables.

4.   6Ethical considerations

The research was analysed and approved by Unochapecó's Human Research Ethics Committee.

The Certificate of Submission for Ethical Appraisal (CAAE) is registered on the Brazil Platform under the number: 48521715.0.0000.0116 (ANNEX III).

The Pittsburgh Sleep Quality Index questionnaire (APPENDIX I), as well as the individual data protocol for each participant (APPENDIX I), were applied after the parents or guardians had completed the Informed Consent Form (ICF) (APPENDIX II).

The questionnaire was administered by means of a declaration of knowledge and agreement from the institutions involved (ANNEX II).

CHAPTER 5

RESULTS

Of the 276 subjects included in the survey, 170 (61.59%) were female. The majority of those interviewed were students in the second year of secondary school (53.99%), followed by the third year (32.97%). The first year had the lowest number of participants (13.04%). The average age was 16.23 ($\pm$ 0.91

years), with the lowest age being 14, represented by a single student, and the highest age recorded being 19, represented by two students.

Two other questions were added to the Pittsburgh Sleep Quality Index, which were deemed necessary to complement the study. The questions are subjective in nature, taking into account each student's personal perception of the characteristics of their sleep, addressing issues such as staying up late and the need to wake up earlier than their peers.

The majority of teenagers (74.91%) reported staying up late to surf the internet, play video games, watch films or series, study or do other activities. This, as already mentioned, is one of the personal and subjective variables, and the concept can vary between individuals, i.e. while one student considers it late to sleep around 11pm, another may consider it early.

The other added question was about the need to wake up earlier than other classmates because they live a long way from their school, in remote neighbourhoods or communities in the countryside. The data collected from the students' responses showed that 82.25 per cent of them slept less than eight hours a night during the month prior to the data collection date, while only 17.75 per cent usually slept more than eight hours (Figure 1).

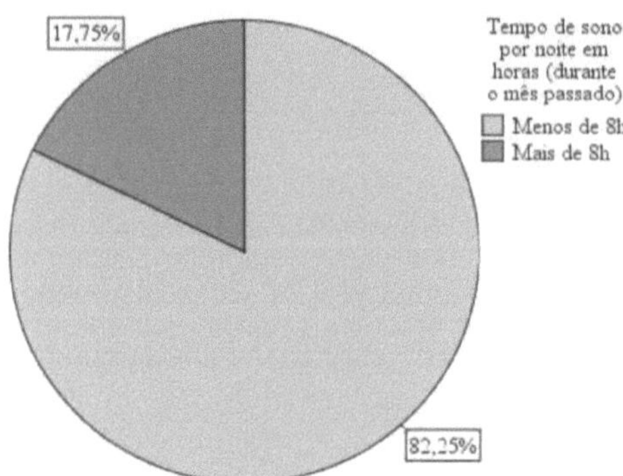

Figure 1 - Hours of sleep per night during the month prior to the data collection date (N=276).

First-year students slept an average of 7.17 (± 1.38) hours a night, second-year students 6.54 (± 1.24) hours, while the average for third-year students was 6.34 (± 1.18) hours a night. With this information, we suspected a possible progressive decline in hours of sleep as the school years progressed, but no statistical significance was found to confirm this hypothesis (p=0.08 between first and second year, p=0.216 between second and third year).

In the questionnaire, the students made a self-assessment of their sleep quality through a question that asked them to classify their sleep in one of the following categories: good, very good, bad or very bad. The majority (57.34%) considered their quality of sleep to be good. No statistically significant difference was found between the grade of secondary school and the self-assessment of sleep quality (p=0.634) (Table 1).

Table 1 - Self-assessment of sleep quality according to secondary school grade (N=276).

Sleep quality	Secondary school grade		
	First year	Second year	Third year
	f(%)	f(%)	f(%)
Very bad	4(1,44)	7 (2.53)	7 (2,53)
Bad	12 (4,34)	28 (10,14)	12 (4,34)
Good	17 (6,15)	71 (25,70)	37 (13,40)
Very good	3 (1)	13 (4,71)	7 (2,53)

f (%): frequency expressed as an absolute number and as a percentage.

The individuals in the survey answered a question about the average time it took them to fall asleep in the last 30 days. The data was grouped into categories ranging from zero to 30 minutes, as well as the category that includes those who reported taking more than 30 minutes to fall asleep. This revealed that 162 (58.70 per cent) students needed more than ten minutes to fall asleep (Table 2).

Table 2 - Time taken to fall asleep during the last month in minutes (N=276).

Time to fall asleep	f (%)
0 to 5 minutes	59 (21,40)
6 to 10 minutes	55 (19,92)
11 to 15 minutes	41 (14,86)
16 to 20 minutes	20 (7.24)
21 to 25 minutes	7 (2,53)
26 to 30 minutes	55 (19,92)
More than 30 minutes	39 (14,13)

f (%): frequency expressed as an absolute number and as a percentage.

The students were asked about their napping habits and then about their intentions. The second question, regarding intentionality, was to be answered only by those who answered "yes" to the question about napping. Among the 181 (65.58%) individuals who reported having the habit of napping, 31.50% of them reported that napping was not an intentional act (Table 3).

Table 3 - Relationship between the act of napping and its intentionality (N=276).

Habit of napping	Number of students f (%)	Intentionality of the napping habit f (%)	
Yes	181 (65,58%)	Yes	124 (68,50%)
		No	57 (31,50%)
No	95 (34,42%)		

f (%): frequency expressed as an absolute number and as a percentage.

In order to answer the question of whether they find it difficult to stay awake during daily activities, the student had to choose one of four alternatives:

not at all, less than once a week, once or twice a week, three times a week or more, always in relation to the 30 days prior to the collection date. Among the individuals who reported sleeping less than eight hours a night, 41 (18.06%) said they had problems staying awake during the day three times a week or more (Figure 2).

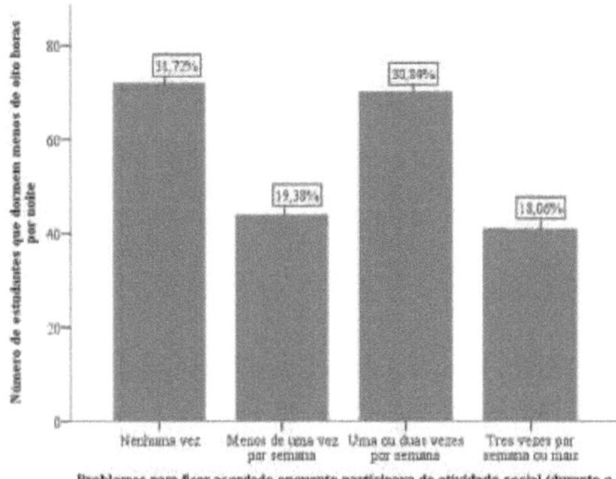

Figura 2 - Relationship between students sleeping less than 8 hours and having problems staying awake (n = 227).

Among the 49 students who reported getting an average of more than eight hours of sleep a night, only five of them (10.20 per cent) indicated that they find it difficult to stay awake during the day at least three times a week or more (Figure 3).

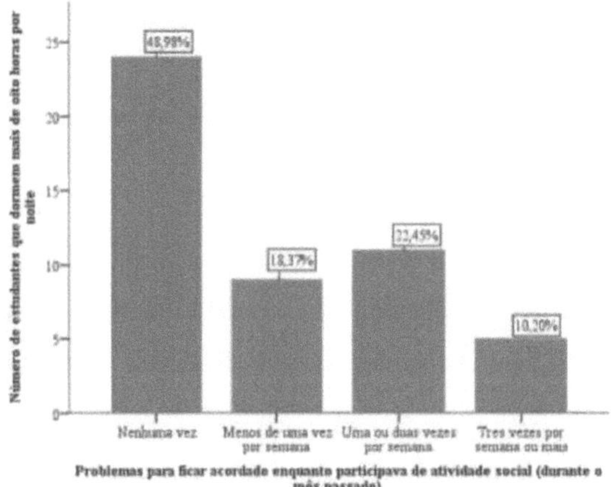

Figura 3   - Relationship between students who sleep more than 8 hours and problems staying awake (n = 49)

When comparing the frequency of problems staying awake between the two groups mentioned above, no statistical significance was found (p=0.115).

However, the average number of hours of sleep for those who had no problem staying awake during the day was 6.98 (± 1.18) hours. The average for those who had trouble staying awake three days a week or more was 6.25 (± 1.25) hours. In other words, there was a decline, albeit modest, in the sleep time of those who reported frequent problems staying awake (three times or more) compared to those who did not identify this difficulty. This comparison proved to be statistically significant (p=0.01).

The students were asked about their use of medication to sleep. We found that 6.60 per cent sought some kind of medication in order to fall asleep. Of these, 16.60 per cent used it less than once a week, 61.10 per cent once or twice a week and 22.30 per cent three times a week or more. In evaluating the answers obtained, any type of medication described was considered valid, as the intention was to check whether there was a search for some artificial means to get to sleep, and not just to find out the pharmacological nature of this medication. Thus, the drugs mentioned ranged from anti-allergic and analgesic drugs (in cases where the adolescent was not sleeping due to some kind of pain), such as Paracetamol® and Dorlfex®, to herbal medicines, i.e. the results were not restricted to hypnotics. Only two (0.72%) of the interviewees reported having used benzodiazepines during the period analysed.After calculating the seven components of the PSQI, it was possible to stratify the individuals in the survey into three groups according to sleep quality. Most of the students (69.20 per cent) had a qualitative sleep pattern classified as poor, i.e. they scored between five and 10 points (Figure 4).

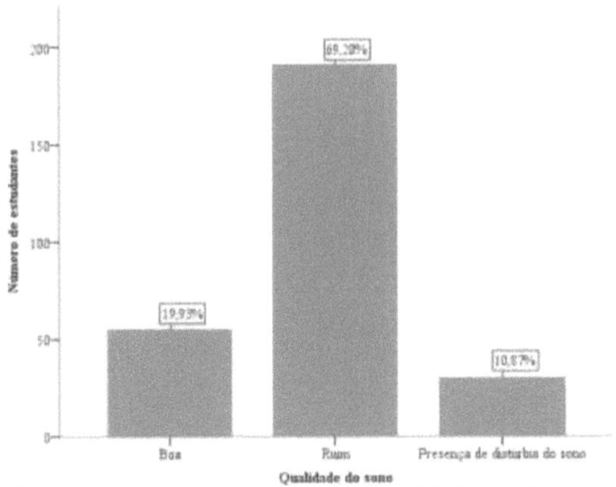

Figure 4 - Relationship between the number of students and sleep quality (N = 276).

After obtaining the results calculated by the PSQI, it was possible to make comparisons between the three high school grades, as well as observe the differences between males and females, in order to verify the particularities and variations in the quality of the sleep-wake cycle of these groups. It emerged that among the individuals who were classified as having sleep disorders, the highest prevalence was found among female students in the third year of secondary school, where nine of them (3.26 per cent) reached the score required to be classified as having sleep-wake cycle disorders. Meanwhile, the highest rate of "bad sleepers", i.e. participants with poor sleep quality, was found among female students in the second year of secondary school.

However, no statistically significant difference was found between the sex of the student and sleep quality (p=0.707) (Figure 5) or between the grade of secondary school and sleep quality (p=0.644) (Figure 6).

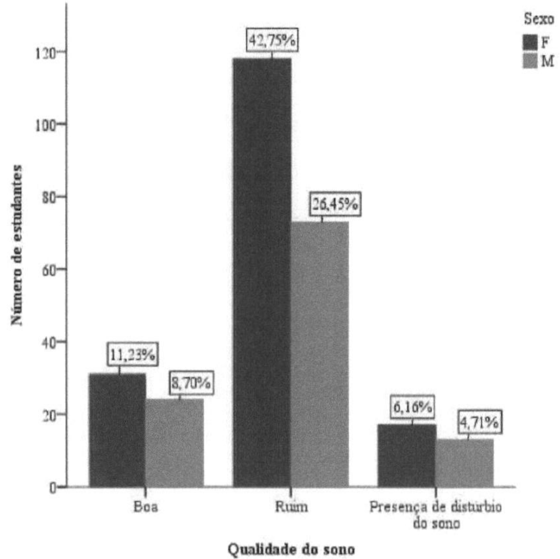

Figure 5 - Relationship between sleep quality and student gender (N = 276).

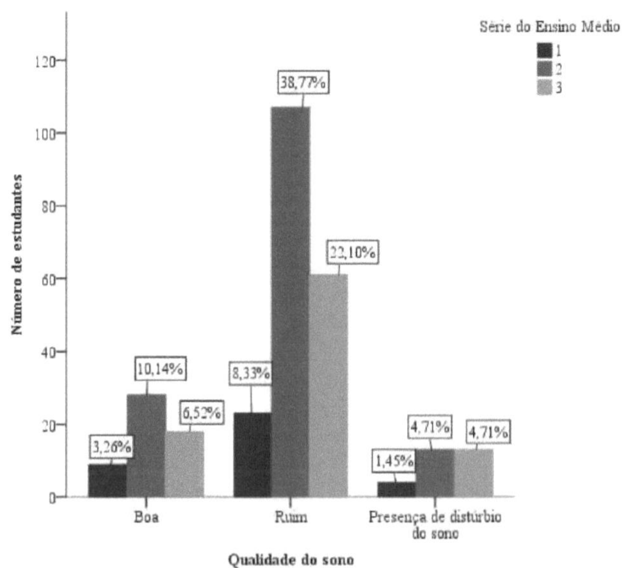

Figure 6 - Relationship between sleep quality and the student's grade (N = 276).

To better visualise and compare the gender and grade variables in relation to sleep quality, the table below was created (Table 4).

Table 4: Classification of sleep quality according to grade and gender (N = 276).

		Sleep quality		
		Good	**Bad**	**Sleep disorder**
Series	**Sex**			
		f (%)	*f* (%)	*f* (%)
First year	F	5 (1,81)	12 (4,35)	2 (0,72)
	M	4 (1,45)	11 (3,98)	2 (0,72)
Second year	F	14 (5,07)	67 (24,30)	6 (2,17)
	M	14 (5,07)	40 (14,49)	7 (2,54)
Third year	F	12 (4,35)	39 (14,13)	9 (3,26)
	M	6 (2,17)	22 (7,97)	4 (1,45)

f (%): frequency expressed in absolute number and percentage. F: Female M: Male

In relation to the nine possible problems that can disrupt the sleep-wake cycle presented by the PSQI, the most prevalent was "taking more than 30 minutes to fall asleep". Only 26 per cent of the adolescents surveyed reported not having had this difficulty during the month prior to the collection date. Two other problems that were also frequent were: "waking up in the middle of the night or very early in the morning" and "feeling too hot". Both were not experienced by only 28.60 per cent of the students (Table 5).

<u>**Table 5: Relationship between sleeping problems and their prevalence (N = 276)**</u>

	Frequency of the problem	Not once	Less than once a week	Once or twice a week	Three times per week or more
Trouble sleeping (over the past month)		f(%)	f(%)	f(%)	f(%)
Taking more than 30 minutes to fall asleep		72 (26)	41 (15)	98 (35,50)	65 (23,50)
Waking up in the middle of the night or very early in the morning		79 (28,60)	42 (15,30)	84 (30,40)	71 (25,70)
Feeling very hot		79 (28,60)	53 (19,20)	121 (43,90)	23 (8,30)
Having bad dreams or nightmares		108 (39,60)	54 (19,80)	80 (29,30)	31 (11,30)
Feeling very cold		118 (45)	45 (17,20)	81 (31)	18 (6.80)
Feeling pain		149 (57,70)	40 (15,50)	53 (20,50)	16 (6,30)
Getting up to go to the toilet		155 (56,10)	45 (16,30)	52 (18,90)	24 (8,70)
Difficulty breathing		206 (74,60)	25 (9)	32 (11,60)	13 (4,80)
Coughing or snoring		223 (81)	17 (6,20)	29 (10,60)	6 (2,20)

f(%): frequency expressed as an absolute number and as a percentage.

CHAPTER 6

DISCUSSION

It was found that a portion of the students (23.5 per cent) slept less than six hours a night in the 30 days preceding the data collection date. Others (25.70 per cent) reported having problems sleeping because they woke up in the middle of the night on three or more days of the week. This is in line with the results presented during the XVI National Sleep Conference, held in France in March 2016, in which a survey of French secondary school students showed that 1/4 of the students slept less than six hours a night and 15% woke up during the night (MIETLICKY, 2016). This is alarming, given that sleep is recognised as being important for quality of life and for preventing mental, physical and psychological illnesses (RIOS; PEIXOTO; SENRA, 2008).

This study expected to find a decrease in the average number of hours of sleep in the more advanced grades. However, although the average number of hours of sleep showed an apparent decrease as the grades progressed, this information was not statistically significant enough to confirm this hypothesis. However, it is important to emphasise that the average amount of sleep per night among the students in the three grades was below the minimum eight hours required for an adolescent suggested by Carskadon (1980, apud PEREZ, 2007).

A study carried out by Pereira et al. (2015) in two cities in southern Brazil, which also targeted adolescent public school students, including university students, showed that the average sleep duration among adolescents with excessive daytime sleepiness (EDS) was 7.9 hours, while for those without excessive daytime sleepiness it was 8.3 hours. This is another piece of information that highlights the relevance of this study, given that more than 82 per cent of the participants reported sleeping less than eight hours a night.

With regard to self-assessment of sleep quality, the study found ambiguity in the adolescents' responses, since when asked to rate their sleep, more than half (57.34%) classified their sleep as good. However, calculating the PSQI score showed that 69.20 per cent of the population studied had a sleep quality classified as poor. A study carried out by Santos (2013) in Portugal also invited adolescent students to self-assess their sleep cycle. The results were similar to the present study, showing that the majority

(54.30%) thought they had a good quality of sleep.

However, in the same Portuguese study, most of the students who said they slept well or even very well felt that they didn't get enough sleep each night. This information brings us back to the survey in question, in which 30.84 per cent of teenagers who said they slept less than eight hours found it difficult to stay awake during the day on at least three days of the week.

One of the main diagnostic criteria for Insomnia Disorder is the presence of difficulty initiating sleep (BACELAR; PINTO JUNIOR, 2013). According to the DSM-V, difficulty in reconciling sleep is defined by a subjective latency period of more than 20-30 minutes. A study carried out in the interior of the state of São Paulo with students from the three grades of secondary school showed that 10.9 per cent of them took more than 30 minutes to fall asleep (MATHIAS; SANCHEZ; ANDRADE, 2006). This figure is similar to the results obtained in the research carried out in Chapecó, in which 14.13 per cent of students reported taking, on average, more than 30 minutes to fall asleep.

In addition to the delay in falling asleep, the DSM-V also includes within the diagnostic criteria for Insomnia Disorder difficulty maintaining sleep, characterised by frequent awakenings or problems returning to sleep after awakening. In our study, the adolescents had to answer a question about waking up in the middle of the night or very early in the morning, and the result was that more than half of them (56.10 per cent) faced this problem at least once a week.

A population-based study carried out in Norway, only with adolescents, calculated the incidence of Insomnia Disorder in this population, according to the DSM-V diagnostic criteria. The result was that 18.50 per cent of that population met the criteria for a diagnosis of insomnia disorder (HYSING et al., 2013). Halbower and Marcus (2003, apud ROCHA; ROSSINI; REIMAO, 2010) report that the prevalence of insomnia among adolescents is approximately 2.2% to 17%, which is in line with the Norwegian study.

This information reaffirms the results found in our study, as the main symptoms related to insomnia showed significant and noteworthy rates. Therefore, it can be concluded that insomnia is a common disorder in adolescence. With regard to this discussion, it is important to note that the First Brazilian Consensus on Insomnia (2002), drawn up by the Brazilian Sleep Society, pointed to a prevalence of 30% to 50% of this sleep disorder in the general population. Currently, the WHO estimates that 40 per cent of Brazilians suffer from some form of insomnia.

In our study, sleep latency was addressed on two occasions, in one of which, as mentioned above, 14.13% of the students reported taking more than 30 minutes to fall asleep. However, when asked again about a series of factors that could disrupt the sleep cycle, 74 per cent of those interviewed claimed to have already had problems sleeping because it took them more than half an hour to fall asleep, at least in a single episode during the 30 days prior to the date of the interview. What changed in this second question about sleep latency was that the participants had to answer the question according to how often the symptom appeared. In this case, 23.50 per cent of the adolescents reported having experienced this difficulty more than three times a week.

Among this series of factors that could disrupt the sleep cycle, the main one presented by the participants in this study was taking more than 30 minutes to fall asleep. This result is similar to that found in two other studies (ROCHA; ROSSINI; REIMAO, 2010) (DUARTE, 2007).

It was found that 65.58 per cent of the study population had the habit of napping. Adolescents have a physiological tendency to sleep and wake up later, but school activities require them to wake up early. As a result, there is a reduction in the number of hours of sleep per night, which is usually compensated for by naps. A result similar to that found in our research was evidenced in a study of third grade high school students in the city of Natal-RN, in which 64% of them had the habit of napping (GUIMARÃES; AZEVEDO, 2009).

In our study, we stratified the individuals into three groups according to their PSQI score. Our sample revealed that 19.93 per cent had good sleep quality (score less than five), 69.20 per cent had poor sleep quality (score between five and 10) and 10.87 per cent had a sleep disorder (score greater than 10). Similar studies have stratified individuals into just two categories: good sleepers (score less than five) and poor sleepers (score greater than five). If we stratify our study in this way, we will have 19.93% of good sleepers and 80.07% of bad sleepers.

A study carried out by Duarte (2007), with a sample of 160 adolescents, found a prevalence of 66.25% of bad sleepers and 33.75% of good sleepers. Another study carried out by Araújo et al. with 600 students from different age groups at the Federal University of Ceará (UFC) found that 50.30 per cent of bad sleepers were in the 16-20 age group. Rocha, Rossoni and Reimão, in a study also carried out only with public school students, found a prevalence of 71.40 per cent of poor sleepers. The latter is the most similar to the result found in this study. However, all of the above-mentioned studies suggest that more than half of adolescents fall into the category of "bad sleepers".

Another study similar to the one presented here was carried out in 1984 with 277 adolescents. The conclusion was that 66 per cent were good sleepers, 23 per cent were occasional poor sleepers and 11 per cent were chronic poor sleepers. This data shows the notable difference between the quality of sleep of the current generation and that of the 1980s, concluding that the quality of sleep of adolescents has deteriorated dramatically over the years.

Based on this comparison, it was possible to consider hypotheses for such a discrepant increase in teenage rough sleepers. In the 1980s there were still no tablets, smartphones or the internet, which was created in 1969 and was for the use of only a few people. The questionnaire applied in our survey revealed that 74.91% of students stay up late to surf the internet, play video games, watch films or series, study or do other activities. From this, we can see the direct interference of these means of leisure on the sleep of adolescents of the current generation.

Bulck (2004) carried out a study in Belgium with 2,546 children to investigate the relationship between the presence of the internet, computers and video games in the bedroom and sleep disorders. The study revealed that the use of electronic devices, especially computers, causes disturbances in sleep patterns, such as going to bed later and waking up later.

According to Duarte (2007), the habit of staying up late at night in front of the computer delays or even shifts sleep from the night to the day, which has repercussions on behaviour during the day. In this context, the present study assessed the presence of difficulties in staying awake while carrying out daily activities. A relationship (p=0.01) was found between the existence of problems staying awake and reduced hours of sleep.

As for sleep quality, no significant relationship was found between gender, grade and the presence of a sleep disorder, which is similar to the data found in the literature (ROCHA; ROSSINI; REIMÃO, 2010). With this information, we can infer that the adolescent population is, in general, sleeping poorly, regardless of gender and secondary school grade.

CHAPTER 7

CONCLUSIONS

This study found that poor sleep quality is a constant among the young people who took part in the research, since 80.07% of them had a result that placed them in the category of "bad sleepers", according to the PSQI. In addition, 74.91 per cent of the adolescents reported staying up late at night to use electronic devices.

It was also observed that there was no significant relationship between the level of education and/or gender of the individuals and the prevalence of sleep disorders. This, together with the high rate of poor sleep quality, shows that the bad habits of

adolescents are equally widespread among age groups and do not distinguish between sexes.

Sleep disorders among adolescents are a real problem and one that deserves attention from parents, educators and the medical community in general, since, according to what was shown in our study, the rates of sleep-wake cycle disorders in the population of adolescent high school students in Chapecó reached the mark of 10.87 per cent of the total number of participants in the study.

The studies in the literature that deal with issues related to sleep disorders still lack depth when it comes to the prevalence of these illnesses among the adolescent population. In addition to being very old, the epidemiological data found is not very precise and is therefore inconclusive.

It can be concluded that this study is relevant not only because of the scarcity of data in relation to the adolescent age group, but also as a tool to alert the population to the importance of good sleep habits.

Having regular bedtimes and wake-up times, going to bed only at bedtime and having an appropriate sleep environment are some of the habits that make for good sleep hygiene. This has a positive impact on the physical and cognitive development of young people, as well as reducing the risks posed by chronic sleep deprivation.

CHAPTER 8

REFERENCES

ADDAMS, Reymond; ROPPER, Allan; VICTOR, Maurice. Principles of Neurology. 7. ed. [s.l.]: Mcgraw-hill, 2000. Chap. 19. p. 199-210.

ADDAMS, Reymond; ROPPER, Allan; VICTOR, Maurice. **Sleep and its abnormalities**. in:
ALMONDES, Katie Moraes de; ARAUJO, John Fontenele de. Pattern of the sleep-wake cycle and its relationship with anxiety in university students. **Estud, Psicol,** Natal, v. 8, n. 1, p. 37-43, Apr. 2003.

ALOE, Flávio; AZEVEDO, Alexandre Pinto de; HASAN, Rosa. Mechanisms of the sleep-wake cycle. **Rev. Bras. Psiquiatr,** São Paulo, v. 27, supl. 1, p. 33-39, mai 2005.

ALVES, Rosana Souza Cardoso; EJZENBERG, Bernardo; OKAY, Yassuhiko. Review of sleep disorders with excessive movement, insomnia and sleepiness in children. **Pediatrics**, São Paulo, v. 24, n. 1, p. 50-64, jan. 2002.

AMERICAN ACADEMY OF SLEEP DISORDERS. **The international classification of sleep disorders, revised**. Chicago, 2001. 401 p.

AMERICAN ACADEMY OF SLEEP MEDICINE. **The AASM Manual for the Scoring of Sleep and Associated Events: Rules, Terminology and Technical Specifications**. Westchester, 2007. 59 p.

AMERICAN PSYCHIATRY ASSOCIATION. **Diagnostic and Statistical Manual of Mental disorders - DSM-5**. 5th ed. Washington: American Psychiatric Association, 2013. 976 p.

ANTUNES, Joaquina; FERNANDES, Pedro; SILVEIRA, Alzira. **"I'm always sleepy, is it a disease?"** - Clinical case of narcolepsy in adolescence. **Scientia Medica,** Porto Alegre, v. 24, n. 1, p. 79-84, 2013.

ARAÚJO, Márcio Flávio Moura de et al. Evaluation of sleep quality among university students in Fortaleza-CE. **Texto & contexto**; Enfermagem, Florianópolis, v.

22, n. 2, p.352-360, jun. 2013.

BACELAR, Andrea; PINTO JUNIOR, Luciano Ribeiro. III Brazilian Consensus on Insomnia. São Paulo: Omnifarma, 2013. 160 p.

BALBANI, A. P. S.; FORMIGONI, G. G. S.. Snoring and obstructive sleep apnoea syndrome. **Rev Ass Med Brasil,** São Paulo, v. 45, n. 3, p. 273-278, jul. 1999.

BEIJAMINI, Felipe. **Evaluation of the sleep/wake cycle, daytime sleepiness and psychomotor performance in adolescents undergoing a sleep education programme.** 2008. 91 f. Dissertation (Master's) - Course in Cellular and Molecular Biology, Federal University of Paraná, Curitiba, 2008.

BERNARDO, Maria Perpeto S. L. et al. Sleep duration in adolescents of different socioeconomic levels. **J. Bras. Psiquiatr,** Rio de Janeiro, v. 58, n. 4, p. 231-237, dec. 2009.

BERTOLAZI, Alessandra Naimaier. **Translation, cultural adaptation and validation of two sleep assessment instruments: Epworth Sleep School and Pittsburgh Sleep Quality Index.** 2008. 93 f. Dissertation (Master's Degree) - Medicine Course, Federal University of Rio Grande do Sul, Porto Alegre, 2008.

BITTENCOURT, Lia Rita Azeredo et al. General approach to patients with obstructive sleep apnoea syndrome. **Rev Bras Hipertens.** Rio de Janeiro, v.16, n. 3, p. 158-163. 2009.

BOSCOLO, Rita A. et al. Evaluation of sleep pattern, physical activity and cognitive functions in school adolescents. **Revista Portuguesa de Ciências do Desporto,** Porto, v. 7, n. 1, p.18-25, Apr. 2007.

BUYSSE, Daniel J. et al. Clinicians' use of the international classification of sleep disorders: results of national survey. Sleep. Pittsburgh, v. 26, n. 1, p. 48-51, sep. 2003.

BUYSSE, Daniel J. et al. The Pittsburgh Sleep Quality Index: A new instrument for psychiatric practice and research. **Psychiatr Research,** Pittsburgh, v. 28, n. 2, p. 193213, mai 1989.

CABRAL, Ana Sofia et al. Narcolepsy, about a clinical case. **Revista de Psiquiatria Consiliar e de Ligação,** Coimbra, v. 16, n. 1, p. 29-37, 2009.

CARDOSO, Hígor Chagas et al. Evaluation of sleep quality in medical students. **Rev. bras. educ. med,** Rio de Janeiro, v. 33, n. 3, p. 349-355, Sep. 2009.

CHELLAPPA, Sarah Laxhmi. Excessive daytime sleepiness and depression: causes, clinical implications and therapeutic management. **Rev. psiquiatr. Rio Gd. Sul,** Porto Alegre, v. 31, n. 3, p. 0-0, 2009.
CIAMPO, Luis Antonio Del. Sleep in adolescence. **Adolesc Saude**, Rio de Janeiro, v.9, n.1, p. 60-66. 2012.

COELHO, Fernando Morgadinho S. et al. Literature Review - Narcolepsy. **Rev. Psiq. Clín,** São Paulo, v. 34, n. 3, p. 133-138, 2007.

CRUZ, Cássio D. Kirchner; SILVA, Cristiana de Camargo e. **Sleep-wake cycle disorders in medical and nursing professionals and students**. 2011. 51 f. TCC (Graduation) - Medicine Course, Universidade Comunitária da Região de Chapecó, Chapecó, 2011.

DUARTE, Gema Galgani de Mesquita. **Sleep quality, school performance and stress in adolescents who spend the night in front of a computer**. 2007. 271 f. Dissertation (Master's) - Medicine Course, State University of Campinas, Campinas, 2007

ENES, Carla Cristina; SLATER, Betzabeth. Obesity in adolescence and its main determinants. **Rev Bras Epidemiol,** São Paulo, v. 13, n. 1, p. 163171, mar. 2010.

FERNANDES, Regina Maria França. Normal sleep. **Medicina,** Ribeirão Preto, v. 39, n. 2, p.157-168, Não é um mês valido! 2006.

FINIMUNDI, Márcia et al . Validation of the circadian rhythm scale - wake/sleep cycle for adolescents. **Rev. Paul. Pediatr.,** São Paulo, v. 30, n. 3, p. 409414, Sep. 2012.

GAINA, Alexandru et al. Daytime sleepiness and associated factors in Japanese school
children. **The Journal Of Pediatrics**, Cincinnati, v. 151, n. 5, p. 518-522, Aug. 2007.

GIBSON, Edward S et al. "Sleepiness" is serious in adolescence: two surveys of 3235 Canadian students. **Bmc Public Health**, London, v. 6, n. 116, p. 1-9, May 2006.

GIORELLI, André S. et al. Excessive daytime sleepiness: clinical, diagnostic and therapeutic aspects. **Rev. Bras. Neurol,** Rio de Janeiro, v. 48, n. 3, p. 17-24, jul-ago-sept. 2012.

GUIMARÃES, Ivanise C. de S.; AZEVEDO, Carolina V. M. de. **A characterisation of knowledge about sleep and the sleeping habits of adolescents**. 2009. 10 f. Psychology Course, Department of Physiology, Federal University of Rio Grande do Norte, Natal - RN, 2009.

HYSING, Mari et al. Sleep patterns and insomnia among adolescents: a population-based study. **J Sleep Res.**, Bergen, Norway, v. 22, p.549-556, mar. 2013.

KIRMIL-GRAY, Kathleen et al. Sleep disturbance in adolescents: Sleep quality, sleep habits, beliefs about sleep, and daytime functioning. **Journal Of Youth And Adolescence**, [s.l.], v. 13, n. 5, p.375-384, nov. 1984.

KLEITMAN, Nathaniel. **Sleep and Wakefulness**. Chicago: Midway Reprint, 1987.

LIU, Xianchen et al. Sleep Patterns and Problems Among Chinese Adolescents. **Paediatrics**. Cincinnati, v. 121, n. 6, p. 1165-1173, jun. 2008.

LOUZADA, Fernando. Et al. The adolescence sleep phase delay: causes, consequences and possible interventions. **Sleep Science**. São Paulo, v. 1, p. 49-53, Oct-Nov-Dec. 2008.

LOUZADA, Fernando; BARRETO, Luiz Silveira Menna. **Biological clocks and learning**. São Paulo: Edesplan, 2004.

MATHIAS, A., SANCHEZ, R. P., ANDRADE, M. M. Encouraging adequate sleep habits: a challenge for educators. **Unesp teaching centre.** São Paulo: Universidade Estadual Paulista, p. 718-731, 2006.

MIETLICKY, Fanny. The sommeil of adolescents, effects of self-portable devices. In: 16ÉME JOURNÉE DU SOMMEIL, 03., 2016, Clamart. **Conference on adolescent sleep, the effects of self-portrait devices**. Clamart: Intitut National Du Sommeil Et de La Vigilance, 2016.

MOREIRA, Gustavo Antonio. Recommendations: Updating Conducts in Paediatrics. **Spsp Scientific Departments.** São Paulo, n. 47, p. 07-14. 2009.

MÚLLER, Mônica R.; GUIMARÃES, Suely S. Impact of sleep disorders on daily functioning and quality of life. **Estudos de Psicologia,** Campinas, v. 24, n. 4, p. 519-528, Oct-Dec. 2007.

NEVES, Gisele S. Moura L. et al. Sleep disorders: an overview. **Revista Brasileira de Neurologia,** Rio de Janeiro, v. 49, n. 2, p. 57-71, Apr-May-Jun. 2013.

NUNES, Magda Lahorgue. Sleep disorders. **Jornal de Pediatria,** Rio de Janeiro, v. 78, n. 1, p. 63-72. 2002.
NUNES, Magda Lahorgue; CAVALCANTE, Verônica. Clinical evaluation and management of insomnia in paediatric patients. **Jornal de Pediatria**, Rio de Janeiro, p. 277-286, Jan. 2005.

PEREIRA, Érico F. et al. Sleep and adolescence: how many hours do adolescents need to sleep? **J. Bras. Psiquiatr.,** Rio de Janeiro, v. 64, n.1, p.40-44, mar. 2015.

PEREIRA, Érico F. et al. Excessive daytime sleepiness in adolescents: prevalence and associated factors. **Rev. Paul. Pediat.,** São Paulo, v. 28, n. 1, p. 98-103, mar. 2010.

PEREZ-CHADA, Daniel et al. Sleep Disordered Breathing And Daytime Sleepiness Are Associated With Poor Academic Performance In Teenagers. A Study Using The Paediatric Daytime Sleepiness Scale (PDSS). **Sleep,** Danvers, v. 30, n. 12, p. 16981703, dec. 2007.

PETROV, Megan E.; LICHSTEIN, Kenneth L.; BALDWIN, Carol M. Prevalence of sleep disorders by sex and ethnicity among older adolescents and emerging adults: Relations to daytime functioning, working memory and mental health. **Journal Of Adolescence,** [s.l.], v. 37, n. 5, p. 587-597, jul. 2014.

RECHTSCHAFFEN, Allan; KALES, Anthony. **A manual of standardised terminology, techniques and scoring system for sleep stages of human subjects.** Los Angeles: Brain Information Service/brain Research Institute, 1968. 59 P.

RIOS, Alaíde Lílian Machado; PEIXOTO, Maria de Fátima Trindade; SENRA, Vani Lúcia Fontes. **Sleep disorders, quality of life and psychological treatment.** 2008. 53 f. TCC (Graduation) - Psychology Course, Faculty of Human and Social Sciences, Vale do Rio Doce University, Governador Valadares, 2008.

ROCHA, Célia R.S.; ROSSINI, Sueli; REIMAO, Rubens. Sleep disorders in high school and pre-university students. **Arq. Neuro-Psiquiatr.,** São Paulo, v. 68, n. 6, p. 903-907, dec. 2010.

RODRIGUES, Tiago Rafael L. P. G. **Narcolepsy: from diagnosis to treatment.** 2012, 35 f. Integrated Master's Degree in Medicine, Faculty of Medicine, University of Porto, 2012.

SANTOS, Andreia Filipa dos. **Sleep and academic performance in Portuguese adolescents.** 2013. 101 f. Dissertation (Master's Degree) - Psychology Course, Instituto Superior de Psicologia Aplicada (ISPA), Lisbon, 2013.

SANTOS, Lucas Cardoso et al. Sleep-wake-circadian cycle disorders - A literature review. **Brazilian Journal Of Surgery And Clincai Research,** Ipatinga, v. 7, n. 2, p. 38-43, Aug. 2014.

SANTOS-SILVA, Rogerio et al. Sleep Disorders and Demand for Medical Services: Evidence from a Population-Based Longitudinal Study. **Plos One,** São Paulo, v. 7, n. 2, p. 1-4, feb. 2012.

SÃO PAULO MUNICIPAL HEALTH SECRETARIAT. **Adolescent Health Care Manual.** São Paulo, 2006. 327 p.

BRAZILIAN SLEEP SOCIETY. **I Brazilian Consensus on Insomnia**. São Paulo, 2003. 45 p.

TEIXEIRA, Liliane Reis et al. Work and excessive sleepiness among Brazilian evening high school students: effects on days off. **International Journal Of Occupational And Environmental Health**, Lodz, v. 16, n. 2, p. 172-177, jun. 2010.

TEIXEIRA, Liliane Reis et. al. Sleep and Sleepiness among Working and Non-Working High School Evening Students. **Chronobiology International**, São Paulo, v. 6, n. 1, p. 99-113. 2007.

TIMO-IARIA, Cézar. Historical evolution of the study of sleep. In: TUFIK, Sergio. **Sleep Medicine and Biology**. Barueri: Manole, 2008. Chap. 1. p. 1-6.

TORPHY, Michael J. Classification of sleep disorders. **Neurotherapeutics,** Bethesda, v. 9, n. 4, p. 687-701, Oct. 2012.

TUFIK, Sérgio. **Sleep Medicine and Biology**. 1. ed. Barueri: Manole, 2008. p. 0145.

VALLE, Luiza Elena R. do; VALLE, Eduardo L. do; REIMÃO, Rubens. Sleep and learning. **Rev. Psicopedagogia**, São Paulo, v. 26, n. 80, p. 286-290. 2009.

WANTANABE, Mayumi et al. Association of short sleep duration with weight gain and obesity at 1-year follow-up. **Sleep**, Japan, v. 33, n. 2, p. 475-480. 2010.

ANNEXES

ANNEX I
Monograph - Sleep disorders in high school students from public schools in Chapecó - SC

PITTSBURGH SLEEP QUALITY INDEX

1) During the past month, what time did you go to bed at night most of the time? TIME OF LIE DOWN: : ___

2) During the past month, how long (minutes) did it take you to fall asleep most of the time? HOW MANY MINUTES IT TOOK TO FALL ASLEEP:

3) During the past month, what time did you wake up in the morning most of the time? WAKE-UP TIME::

4) During the past month, how many hours of sleep did you get per night? (This may differ from the number of hours you spent in bed) HOURS OF SLEEP PER NIGHT:

For each of the following questions, choose only one answer that you think is most correct. Please answer all the questions.

5) Over the past month, how often have you had trouble sleeping because of..:

a) Taking more than 30 minutes to fall asleep
( )not once   ( )less than once a week
( )once or twice a week   ( )three times a week or more
b) Waking up in the middle of the night or very early in the morning
( )not once   ( )less than once a week
( )once or twice a week   ( )three times a week or more
c) Getting up to go to the toilet
( )not once   ( )less than once a week
( )once or twice a week   ( )three times a week or more
d) Having difficulty breathing
( )not once   ( )less than once a week
( )once or twice a week   ( )three times a week or more

e) Coughing or snoring loudly
( )not once   ( )less than once a week
( )once or twice a week   ( )three times a week or more

f) Feeling very cold
( )not once   ( )less than once a week
( )once or twice a week   ( )three times a week or more

g) Feeling very hot
( )not once   ( )less than once a week
( )once or twice a week   ( )three times a week or more

h) Having bad dreams or nightmares
( )not once   ( )less than once a week
( )once or twice a week   ( )three times a week or more

i) Feeling pain
( )not once   ( )less than once a week
( )once or twice a week   ( )three times a week or more
j) Any other reason? Please describe: ____

k) How many times have you had trouble sleeping for this reason over the past month?
( )not once   ( )less than once a week
( )once or twice a week   ( )three times a week or more

6) Over the past month, how would you rate the quality of your sleep?
( )Very good   ( )bad
( )Good   ( )very bad

7) During the past month, have you taken any sleeping pills, either prescribed by your doctor or recommended by someone else (pharmacist, friend, family member) or even on your own?
   ( )not once   ( )less than once a week
   ( )once or twice a week   ( )three times a week or more

Which one(s)?

8) During the past month, if you've had trouble staying awake while eating your meals or taking part in any other social activity, how often has this happened?
( )not at all ( )less than once a week
   ( )once or twice a week   ( )three times a week or more

9) During the past month, have you felt unwell or lacking in enthusiasm to carry out your daily activities?

( ) No indisposition or lack of enthusiasm
( ) Little indisposition and lack of enthusiasm
( ) Moderate indisposition and lack of enthusiasm
( ) Very unwell and lacking in enthusiasm

10) Do you doze off?
( )YES ( )NO

11) If so, do you nod off intentionally, i.e. because you want to?
( )YES ( ) NO

12) For you, napping is:
( ) A pleasure
( ) A necessity
( ) Other - which?__________________________________

ANNEX II

DECLARAÇÃO DE CIÊNCIA E CONCORDÂNCIA DAS INSTITUIÇÕES ENVOLVIDAS

Local: *Chapecó, Santa Catarina*

Data: *28 / 07 / 2015*

Com o objetivo de atender às exigências para obtenção de parecer da Comitê de Ética em Pesquisa envolvendo Seres Humanos da Unochapecó, o representante legal da instituição *Carlos Frederico de Almeida Rodrigues* envolvida no projeto de pesquisa intitulado *Distúrbios do Sono em Adolescentes Estudantes do Ensino Médio em Escolas Públicas de Chapecó - SC* declara estar ciente e de acordo com seu desenvolvimento nos termos prepostos, salientando que os pesquisadores deverão cumprir os termos da resolução 466/12 do Conselho Nacional de Saúde.

____
Assinatura do Pesquisador Responsável

Carlos Frederico de Almeida Rodrigues

____
Assinatura e Carimbo do responsável da Instituição

Maria Salete Perin
Supervisora de Educação Superior
Mat. 129.095-9-01

Maria Salete Perin
Supervisora de Educação Superior

ANNEX III

UNIVERSIDADE COMUNITÁRIA DA REGIÃO DE CHAPECÓ- UNOCHAPECÓ

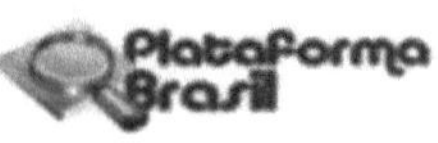

COMPROVANTE DE ENVIO DO PROJETO

DADOS DO PROJETO DE PESQUISA

Título da Pesquisa: DISTÚRBIOS DO SONO EM ESTUDANTES DO ENSINO MÉDIO EM ESCOLAS PÚBLICAS DE CHAPECÓ - SC

Pesquisador: Carlos Frederico

Versão: 2

CAAE: 48521715.0.0000.0116

Instituição Proponente: Universidade Comunitária Regional de Chapecó

DADOS DO COMPROVANTE

Número do Comprovante: 083266/2015

Patrocionador Principal: Financiamento Próprio

Informamos que o projeto DISTÚRBIOS DO SONO EM ESTUDANTES DO ENSINO MÉDIO EM ESCOLAS PÚBLICAS DE CHAPECÓ - SC que tem como pesquisador responsável Carlos Frederico, foi recebido para análise ética no CEP Universidade Comunitária da Região de Chapecó-UNOCHAPECÓ em 24/08/2015 às 16:09.

Endereço: Av. Senador Attilio Fontana, 591 E
Bairro: Efapi   **CEP:** 89.809-000
UF: SC   **Município:** CHAPECO
Telefone: (49)3321-8142   **Fax:** (49)3321-8142   **E-mail:** cep@unochapeco.edu.br

APPENDICES

APPENDIX I

Individual Data Protocol

Question 1 - What grade are you in? ( ) 1st year MS ( ) 2nd year MS ( ) 3rd year MS

Question 2 - How old are you? years

Question 3 -Gender: ( ) Male ( ) Female

Question 4 - Do you usually stay up late to surf the internet, play video games or watch films/series?

        ( ) YES   ( ) NO

Question 5 - Do you have to wake up earlier than your classmates because you live a long way from your school (remote neighbourhoods, rural communities)?

        ( ) YES   ( ) NO

APPENDIX II

COMMUNITY UNIVERSITY OF THE CHAPECÓ REGION - UNOCHAPECÓ
HEALTH SCIENCES - MEDICINE COURSE
GIANCARLOS BRUM FORNARI; GIULIA LUIZA CECCONELLO
TUTOR: CARLOS ALBERTO DO AMARAL MEDEIROS

Consent form

COMMUNITY UNIVERSITY OF THE CHAPECÓ REGION - UNOCHAPECÓ
AREA OF HEALTH SCIENCES
MEDICAL COURSE

INFORMED CONSENT FORM
You are being invited to take part in a research study as a volunteer. If you agree to take part in the study, please sign the two copies at the end of this document. One copy is yours and the other belongs to the researcher.

Project title: SLEEP DISORDERS IN HIGH SCHOOL STUDENTS IN PUBLIC SCHOOLS IN CHAPECÓ - SC

Researcher responsible / Co-supervisor: Carlos Frederico de Almeida Rodrigues
Contact telephone: (54) 91418414
Students: Giancarlos B. Fornari; Giulia L. Cecconello

The aim of this study was to identify the prevalence of sleep-wake cycle disorders in adolescent high school students from public schools in the city of Chapecó-SC.

Your participation in the research consists of answering an interview conducted by the pair of researchers, without any embarrassment or humiliation. The content of the questions poses no risk to your physical or moral integrity. The information collected in the interview will be of great value in achieving the objective mentioned above and in building a discussion on the subject. If, after answering the questionnaire, you no longer wish to take part in the research, please contact us on the telephone number mentioned above.

CONSENT TO THE PARTICIPATION OF THE PERSON AS SUBJECT
Me, ____RG

CPF ___________________ , undersigned, agree to participate in the study as a subject. I have been duly informed and clarified by the researcher   about the research and the procedures involved, as well as

and the benefits of my participation. I was assured that I could withdraw my consent at any time.

Place: ________________________________Date: ___/___/_____ .

Name and   signature of the person responsible:

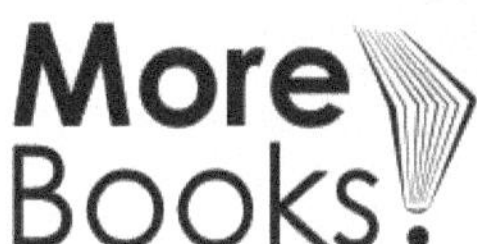

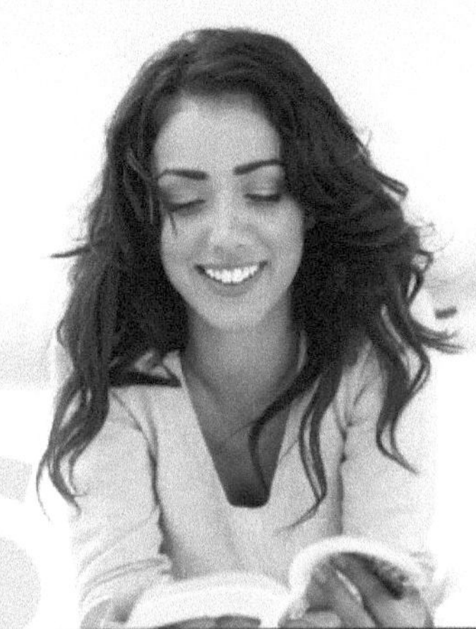

I want morebooks!

Buy your books fast and straightforward online - at one of world's fastest growing online book stores! Environmentally sound due to Print-on-Demand technologies.

Buy your books online at
www.morebooks.shop

Kaufen Sie Ihre Bücher schnell und unkompliziert online – auf einer der am schnellsten wachsenden Buchhandelsplattformen weltweit! Dank Print-On-Demand umwelt- und ressourcenschonend produziert.

Bücher schneller online kaufen
www.morebooks.shop

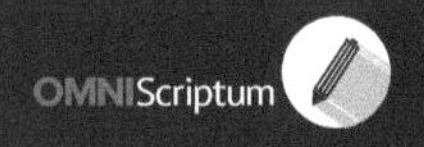